Book 1:
The Beginners Guide to Making Your Own Essential Oils

BY LINDSEY P

&

Book 2:
The Beginners Guide to Medicinal Plants

BY LINDSEY P

Book 1:

The Beginners Guide to Making Your Own Essential Oils

BY LINDSEY P

Complete Guide to Making Your Own Essential Oils from Scratch & To Improve Your Health and Well-Being

ESSENTIAL OILS BOX SET #15: The Beginners Guide to Making Your Own Essential Oils and The Beginners Guide to Medicinal Plants

Table Of Contents

Introduction

I want to thank you and congratulate you for purchasing the book, *The Beginners Guide To Making Your Own Essential Oils: Complete Guide To Making Your Own Essential Oils From Scratch & To Improve Your Health And Well-Being*.

This book contains proven steps and strategies on how to make your very own essentials oils to keep you healthy and away from many diseases and sicknesses.

Since the beginning of time, aromatherapy has been used by our ancestors to promote health, for medical practice and for personal hygiene. Aromatherapy uses essential oils extracted from flowers, stems, leaves, barks and other parts of a plant. These essential oils are believed to enhance physical as well as psychological well-being.

The aroma of these essential oils is believed to stimulate brain function when inhaled. Essential oils are also absorbed through the skin easily, wherein they promote well-being and healing by travelling through the bloodstream.

More and more people are discovering the medicinal benefits of aromatherapy, which is why it is gaining popularity really fast. Aromatherapy is used in various applications including increased cognitive function, enhanced mood and pain relief.

There are numerous essential oils and aromatherapy products available. Each of them has their own healing properties.

This book explains what essential oils are and how they are made. Inside, you will also discover various essential oils and the benefits that they offer. You can use this book as a guide on how to use aromatherapy and which essential oil is best to use for a specific condition.

Thanks again for purchasing this book, I hope you enjoy it!

Chapter 1

What Are Essential Oils

Essential oils are extracted from leaves, flowers, barks, stems, roots and other parts of a plant, commonly by steam. Essential oils are commonly clear but may also have amber, yellow or deep blue color. Essential oils are also referred to as essences since they contain the true essence of the plant where they are extracted from. Although essential oils have pleasing aromatic scents, they are different from fragrance oils.

Unlike fragrance oils, essential oils are pure and do not contain artificial fragrances or substances, that is why fragrance oils are not suitable for aromatherapy. Essential oils are used for its therapeutic benefits since the beginning of recorded history. These essential oils are usually inhaled or applied to the skin for absorption. History has proven the psychological and physical therapeutic benefits of essentials oils, although no scientific evidence has proven it.

Since essential oils are either inhaled or applied directly to the skin, you should take time to check if you have any allergic reactions to any of them. Apply a small amount to the side of your hand and wait for a few hours for any allergic reactions. Moreover, if you are allergic to the source plant, fruit or seed, chances are, you are also allergic to the essential oil extracted from it.

Although they are called "essential oils", they are not really oils. Unlike actual oil, essential oils do not contain fatty acids which make them actual oil. Furthermore, essential oils are volatile and they evaporate when left uncovered. Essential oils are often diluted in carrier oils such as grape seed oil, sweet almond oil and apricot kernel oil. You can buy essential oils individually bottled in small bottles. Most essential oils are sold as blends of various essential oils such as the Thieves essential oil. This essential oil is a combination of clove, lemon, cinnamon, eucalyptus and rosemary essential oils.

Chapter 2

An Easy Way to Make Your Own Essential Oil At Home

Essential oils are generally extracted from plants through distillation, commonly using steam. But other processes are also used such as solvent extraction, florasols extraction and expression. Essential oils are greatly used in perfumes, soaps and cosmetics. They are also used to flavor food and drinks and to add scent to household cleaning products and incense.

One of the most popular and easiest essential oil to make at home is the orange essential oil. Orange peels usually end up in the garbage and are just wasted. Instead of buying expensive scents, you can make your very own citrus scent at home without spending too much. Furthermore, making your own essential oil means you are guaranteed to be using a 100% natural product, free from harmful chemicals.

This procedure is an example of extracting essential oil using alcohol.

All you need are the following:

Orange peels (remove most of the white pith as possible)

Glass jar or glass bottle with a tight lid

Vodka (No need for the expensive ones. Any cheap vodka will do)

Undenatured Ethyl alcohol (as a substitute for the Vodka)

Coffee filter (cheesecloth or muslin will do)

Paper towel (muslin or cheesecloth can also be used as a substitute)

Dry your orange peels in a warm, dry place but away from direct sunlight until they are hard and dry. It usually takes 2 days for this but you can cut the orange peels into smaller pieces to help dry them faster.

Place the dried orange peels into the glass jar or bottle. Place the bottle of vodka or undenatured ethyl alcohol into a bowl of hot tap water for a few minutes then pour it into the jar/bottle of dried orange peels until they are all soaked. Cover the jar/bottle tightly and shake it vigorously for 2 to 3 minutes. Do this three to four times a day for 3 days or more. The more you shake the mixture and the longer you leave the orange peels soaked, the more oil you can extract.

Using a coffee filter or cheesecloth, strain the orange peels into a bowl. Cover it with cheesecloth or paper towel. Do not let the towel/cloth fall into the liquid as it will seep it and you will lose your essential oil.

Let the liquid sit for a few days in a cool, dark and clean area until all the alcohol has evaporated. Now you have pure orange essential oil that you can use for fragrance, soaps, candles, lotion, potpourris or aromatic waters.

When extracting essential oil from leaves or flowers using undenatured ethyl alcohol or vodka, the process is almost the same as above. The only difference is, when you strain the flowers/leaves from the mixture, you need to gently press them to release more oil. Furthermore, while you are soaking them in alcohol or vodka, you can add more leaves or flowers until you are able to reach your desired strength for your essential oil.

Chapter 3

How to Make Your Own Essential Oil At Home through Distillation

The most popular way of extracting essential oil from plants is through distillation. Normally, you need an apparatus called the still to be able to collect essential oil from plants. But, if you do not have distillation equipment and you want to create your own essential, it is still possible. The yield may not be as great as when you are using a still and the process may be longer but it's a great alternative.

You will need a crock pot, some distilled water, air-tight glass container, bowl and cheesecloth. This procedure is very simple but it takes time.

- Decide what plant material you want to extract essential oil from. Dry your plant material. Make sure not to over dry them and do not place them under direct sunlight as it may lose some of its essential oils.

- Place your dried plant material into the crock pot and fill it with distilled water until all the plant material is soaked.

- Cook in low heat for 24 hours. Do not attempt to increase the heat to make the process faster as it will affect the quality and yield of the essential oil.

- Leave crock pot open until cool. Cover with cloth and let it sit in a cool, dry place for a week. You will see oil separating on top of the water in the crock pot. Collect the oil off and place it in a dark, tightly covered container.

- Cover the container with cheesecloth and allow the rest of the water to evaporate. This will take about a week.

- You now have your very own essential oil made possible through distillation at home.

Another distillation method that can be done at home is by grounding up your dried plant material. Use a cotton or linen bag as a container for your ground plant material for cooking. Make sure to tie the bag shut so that no plant material falls off during the process.

Put some distilled water in a crock pot, enough to soak up the bag of plant material. Bring it to a boil. When the water is already boiling, reduce the heat to low and let it simmer for 24 hours.

Let the water cool. You will notice some oil on the surface of the water. Collect the oil and place in a clean, dry, dark glass container. Squeeze the bag unto the water in the crock pot and collect the oil from the surface.

Cover the glass container with clean cloth (cheesecloth or cotton preferably). Let it sit in a cool, dry place for a week to allow the excess water to evaporate.

You can now enjoy your very own essential oil.

Chapter 4

How to Use Oil to Extract Essential Oil

Extracting essential oil using is very and can be done from home. It is most ideal to use almond oil, Jojoba oil or rapeseed for this process. Do not use a metal container when using oils to extract essential oils from plant materials as it will affect the quality of the essential oil. Use non-metallic containers only such as ceramic crock or glass containers.

This process is best used for herbs and flowers such as rosemary, lavender, rose or the likes. You may or may not dry your herb or flowers. It all depends on you. Drying can reduce the amount of essential oil from your herb/flower but it can help increase your yield per batch as you will be able to cramp in more herbs/flowers per batch.

Things you will need:

Large glass bottle

Extracting oil (rapeseed, almond or jojoba)

Cheesecloth

Procedure:

Fill half of the large glass bottle with your extracting oil (carrier oil) such as jojoba, rapeseed or almond). Put as much herbs/flowers/leaves into the glass bottle. Make sure that all the plant materials are completely submerged into the oil. Cover the glass tightly with its lid and let sit for 24 hours in a cool, dark, clean area.

Shake the mixture from time to time within three days. You can do this three to four times each day. Shaking will help extract more oil from the plant material.

After three days, strain the plant material. Use a ceramic bowl to catch the oil from the glass bottle. You can add more plant materials into the oil if the scent is not strong enough for you. Remember, you have to let it sit for 24 hours and repeat all the process after that.

Place your extracted essential oil in a dark, clean container. This essential oil is ready to use.

Another way of extracting essential oil from a plant material using oil is by slow cooking. Here's how to do it:

- In a crock pot, place 2 cups of olive oil (jojoba, rapeseed or almond) and mix ½ ounce of plant material (flowers, leaves, herbs, etc) into it.

- Slow cook the mixture in low heat for up to 6 hours. You may stir the mixture a few times to ensure that the plant materials are completely soaked into the carrier oil (olive oil, jojoba, rapeseed, almond).

- Leave the crock pot open to cool the mixture.

- Strain the oil mixture using an unbleached cheese cloth. Use a ceramic bowl to place the oil while straining.

- Place the essential oil in a dark, clean, tightly covered glass bottle and use sparingly.

Another easy way of extracting essential oil from plant materials using is by grounding the plant materials and soaking them in carrier oils. This process takes a long time of waiting but it's fairly easy to do.

First, dry your plant material. Do not expose your plant material in direct sunlight as it will lose most of its essential oils. Dry in a dark, cool place for about 2 days. Do not over dry. When the plant material is already wilted and dried, it's ready to be grounded.

After grinding the plant material, take one tablespoon and place it in a clear, glass bottle or jar. Add ½ cup of carrier oil (olive oil, rapeseed, almond, jojoba) and ½ teaspoon white vinegar. Stir to combine all the ingredients. Cover the glass bottle/jar and leave it in a warm, sunny area for three weeks. Make sure to place the bottle in an area where there is plenty sunlight. Shake the bottle two to three times a day for three weeks.

Strain the mixture and place your essential oil in a dark, glass container. Please note that essential oils are very pure so they must be used in small amounts only.

To ensure that you are not allergic to any essential oils, perform the skin patch test. Place a small amount of essential oil on the side of your palm. Wait for a few hours. If no irritation, itchiness or swelling occurs, you are not allergic to the essential oil and you may continue using it. In general, if you are allergic to the herb, flower or fruit of a certain plant, you are most likely allergic to its essential oil as well.

Chapter 5

Essential Oils: Uses and Benefits

The use of essential oils and making your own at home can be very fun, fulfilling and beneficial therapeutically. Always remember that essential oils are not meant to be swallowed or ingested. There may be some essential oils that are safe to ingest, but even so, you still need to consult an expert before ingesting any essential oils.

Essential oils are commonly inhaled. For first timers, you can place one to two drops of your desired essential oil in a piece of tissue and carefully inhale the scent. Those who are already veterans in using essential oils usually place a small amount of essential oil on their palm and rub it a little, and then they cover their nose with their palm and inhale the aroma of the essential oil.

When you are suffering from colds or influenza, the best way to treat your condition with essential oils is through steam inhalation. Pour 2 cups of boiled water in a bowl and add 3 to 7 drops of essential oil into it. You may lessen the number of drops if you are using essential oils with strong scents that may irritate your mucus membranes. Some of these essential oils include thyme, rosemary, cinnamon, pine eucalyptus, cajuput and others. Do not place your nose too near the bowl. Put at least about 10 to 12 inches gap between the bowl and your nose. Inhale the steam gradually and carefully. Do not inhale constantly as it may irritate your nose. If you feel any discomfort or irritation, discontinue use right away. This can be done anytime, day or night.

Please note that too much inhalation of essential oils can cause dizziness, vertigo, lethargy, nausea and headaches. Although essential oils are greatly used to treat respiratory problems and sinuses, you must take precaution when using them. Do not use over 10 drops. Aside from hot water, you may also use diffusers or hot compress for inhalation.

Essential oils are also great for making your room smell fresh. To expel any unwanted smell in your house, you may sprinkle a few drops of essential oils in your trash can, drain, vacuum bag filter or laundry wash. You may also add a few drops on your tissue before you keep them in your cabinet. Please take note that essential oils are flammable. Do not place them near fire or too much heat.

Essential oils are also great insect repellents. Essential oils of citronella, peppermint and lavender are natural insect repellents. To prevent insects from infesting your household, place a few drops on a cotton ball and place it on your doorway, windows and other areas where you frequently see insects. If you are a pet owner, some essential oils are not suitable for pets. Some of these essential oils include anise, garlic, juniper, horseradish, clove leaf or clove bud, thyme, Wintergreen, yarrow and others.

On the contrary, there are also some essential oils that are used for pets, especially for dogs due to their calming effects. Most common of these are chamomile, eucalyptus, lavender, ginger, myrrh, rose, valerian, cedarwood atlas, ravensare and others. Essential oils are usually used for pet baths and for calming the pet's nerves through diffusion.

Remember that your pet cannot tell you if it is or is not working. Always check for signs of irritation as excessive scratching, too much whining, sniffing and nervousness. If any of these signs are present, discontinue use.

Either for humans or for pets always dilute your essential oil. For pets, essential oils are best diluted at 25% of human formula. Never use essential oils internally for your pets. Size matters for essential oils. Smaller pets should be given smaller amount of essential oil. But even if your pet is huge, let's say a horse; less is still better with essential oils. Birds and fish should never be given essential oils. Birds are highly sensitive and cannot tolerate essential oils just as fish cannot tolerate floral waters or oils.

Essential oils are also greatly used for a relaxing massage. Do not use any essential oil that is not diluted as it may cause skin irritations. Use 1 ounce of carrier oil such as almond oil and add 10 to 20 drops of essential oil. Do not apply on the genitals and near the eyes.

Essential oils are also popularly used for soaps, shampoos, lotions, shower gels, facial toners and perfumes for their great aroma and therapeutic benefits.

If you are experiencing circulatory problems, skin problems, respiratory symptoms, menstrual pain, muscle pain or stress and nervous tension, an aromatic bath will give you great relief. Please be aware that essential oils should be mixed with either salt or emulsifier like sesame oil or milk before they can be safely dispersed into the water. Essential oils will float on water if not mixed with salt or emulsifier and will directly get into the skin which can cause irritations.

Aromatic bath uses warm water and essential oils that are not mixed with salt or emulsifier can cause dermotoxicity especially if the essential oil used is of a heating nature. For safety purposes, avoid spicy oils in your bath. These essential oils include thyme, tulsi, oregano and cinnamon oil. Also, avoid phototoxic oils such as bergamot oil and citrus oils. Essential oils with specific irritant potential such as lemongrass should also be avoided. Essential oils that are generally considered mild for use in baths are:

- Lavender oil

- Clary Sage oil

- Rose oil

- Geranium oil

- Frankincense oil

- Sandalwood oil

- Eucalyptus oil

- Cedar oil

- Fir oil

- Pine oil

- Pinon pine essential oil

- Spruce oil

- Juniper oil

Combine 5 to 10 drops of essential oil in ½ to 1 cup of salt or emulsifier and add it into your warm bath. Do not soak too long in aromatic water. The ideal soaking time is between 10 to 15 minutes only. Soaking too long under aromatic baths may cause skin irritation and other symptoms such as headache and nausea.

If you suffer from dysmenorrhea or menstrual cramps, skin problems and muscle aches or if you have a wound or a bruise, you can use essential oil (lavender, thieves, Melrose) compress for relief. Just add 10 drops of essential oil in 4oz of warm water and soak a clean cloth in it. Wring the cloth gently and place it on the affected area. Repeat the process for 10 to 15 minutes.

For relief from inflammation, you may use the following essential oils for your compress:

- Wintergreen – This essential oil has a warming effect. Its methyl salicylate and cortisone-like effect reduces inflammation and pain in the muscles and joints.

- Helichrysum – This essential oil has powerful anti-inflammatory properties making it ideal for cuts and bruises. It also helps boost circulation and cleanses the blood.

- Clove – This essential oil helps relieve pain due to arthritis and rheumatism. It has anti-infectious properties as well as anti-inflammatory, anesthetic and antiseptic properties which also make it ideal for wounds, scrapes and bruises.

- Peppermint – For pain, peppermint essential oil is great. It has pain blocking properties, antispasmodic and anti-inflammatory properties. It provides cooling and soothing effects and it also dilates the respiratory system.

- Palo Santo – Due to its anticoagulant and anti-inflammatory properties, this essential oil is excellent for relieving tired muscles and joints. It is also rich in limonene, an antioxidant.

- Lemon – Essential oil extracted from lemon has antiseptic properties which make it great for wounds and cuts. It also has immune-stimulating properties which uplifts your mood.

- Copal/Copaiba – This essential oil has excellent anti-inflammatory properties which are good for wounds, cuts and bruises. It is also an antiseptic, antibacterial and analgesic. Furthermore, Copaiba/Copal essential oil helps boost the respiratory, nervous and cardiovascular systems.

Essential oils are also used for massage due to their calming and warming effects as well as their therapeutic benefits. Take note that essential oils are pure and must be diluted in carrier oils before use. For adults, it is ideal to place 12 drops of essential oil in an ounce of carrier oil. For children under 12 years old, it is generally safe to use 6 drops of essential oil in an ounce of carrier oil. You may lessen the number of drops for the essential oils especially if you are just starting.

Chapter 6

List of Essential Oils and Their Uses

There are so many essential oils out in the market and there are even more that are yet to be discovered. Below is a quick guide to essential oils and their uses.

- Basil – This essential oil is antiviral, antibacterial, antispasmodic and anti-inflammatory. It is also a muscle relaxant, stimulant, decongestant and antiseptic. Due to its therapeutic properties, basil essential oil is often used to treat migraines, muscle aches and pains, mental fatigue, anxiety, depression, throat and lung infections, bronchitis, menstrual cramps, dandruff and insect bites. It can also be used as an insect repellant for flies and mosquitoes.

  You may dilute it in carrier oil such as vegetable or coconut oil. A 50:50 dilution is ideal, meaning one part basil essential oil is to one part carrier oil. You may apply the diluted basil essential oil in the problem areas or inhale it by placing 1 to 2 drops on the palm of your hand rubbing it lightly. If you are asthmatic, do not inhale any essential oil. Instead, place it on the sole of your feet. You may also diffuse it by using the candle method or the steam method.

- Bergamot – Bergamot is known for its relaxing and uplifting effect and has a sweet and fruity scent. It is used to help fight addiction and to relieve stress, anxiety and depression. It is also know to relieve infections such as herpes and vaginal candida as well as cold sores, urinary tract infections and respiratory infections. You may use diluted Bergamot essential oil for massage or apply topically on the affected area. You can also diffuse it or inhale it by adding a few drops on your palm.

- Clary Sage – The sharp, grassy and spicy aroma of Clary Sage essential oil helps relax the mind. It helps prevent hair loss by boosting hair growth. It is an antioxidant, astringent and antiseptic making it effective in preventing wrinkles and keeps skin healthy (for dry and oily skin). It helps relieve menstrual problems and PMS, pre-menopausal symptoms, insomnia, impotence, hemorrhoids, bronchitis, high cholesterol and kidney disorders.

- Chamomile – Chamomile essential oil can tone the skin through continued use. It is also a known anti-depressant and reduces nervousness.

- Cinnamon – For the relief of joint pains and improved circulation, cinnamon essential oil is greatly advised. It also helps reduce nervousness by calming the nerves.

- Cucumber – Essential oil extracted from cucumber is an excellent detoxifier and skin moisturizer. It also helps reduce puffiness of the eyes. The calming effect of cucumber essential oil is great for relaxing the mind and body.

- Eucalyptus – This essential oil is effective in killing lice. Dilute one part eucalyptus essential oil to one part coconut oil and apply to hair. Leave for 5 to 10 minutes only. Rinse off with water or shampoo. It also eases joint and muscle pains and clears respiratory passages.

- Jasmine – This is a must-have for girls. Jasmine essential oil reduces scars and helps relieve PMS symptoms. It is also effective in relieving muscle spasms and for treating dry and sensitive skin.

- Lavender – This essential oil is best known for its calming effect making it an effective treatment for insomnia and stress. It also reduces symptoms of PMS.

- Lemon – Lemon essential oil is known to clear respiratory passages making it effective for the treatment of colds and other respiratory problems. The antibacterial and antiseptic properties of lemon essential oil also make it an effective treatment for acne. It also boosts the immune system, treat dandruff and helps lower down fever.

- Orange – Essential oil from orange has anti-inflammatory properties which relieve pain and inflammation. It is also an anti-depressant and an aphrodisiac.

- Peppermint – For fast relief of headache, peppermint essential oil is highly recommended. It also relieves nausea and decreases indigestion. It also eases clogged nose and relieves other respiratory problems.

- Sage – Sage essential oil heals wounds, fights infections and calms upset stomach.

Always remember to store your essential oils in a cool dry place and away from direct sunlight and heat as it may lose its potency and its quality can be compromised.

Conclusion

Thank you again for purchasing this book!

I hope this book was able to help you learn how to make your own essential oil from scratch and know more about the uses and benefits of essential oils.

The next step is to start making your own essential oils and start living a healthier and stress-free life.

Finally, if you enjoyed this book, please take the time to share your thoughts and post a review on Amazon. We do our best to reach out to readers and provide the best value we can. Your positive review will help us achieve that. It'd be greatly appreciated!

Thank you and good luck!

Book 2:

The Beginners Guide to Medicinal Plants

BY LINDSEY P

Everything You Need to Know About the Healing Properties of Plants & Herbs, How to Grow and Harvest Them

ESSENTIAL OILS BOX SET #15: The Beginners Guide to Making Your Own Essential Oils and The Beginners Guide to Medicinal Plants

Table Of Contents

Introduction

I want to thank you and congratulate you for purchasing the book, *"The Beginners Guide to Medicinal Plants"*.

This book contains proven steps and strategies on how to successfully grow medicinal plants and herbs right at the very comfort of your own home.

Featured in this book are some of the most common mistakes when putting up a medicinal garden at home and how to avoid committing such mistakes. Also featured in this book are some of the best types of medicinal plants to grow at home.

Thanks again for purchasing this book, I hope you enjoy it!

Chapter 1: Guide to Growing a Medicinal Herb Garden

Growing medicinal plants and herbs indoor is a popular hobby for a lot of gardeners. One of the greatest reasons to plant medicinal plants indoor is to have a ready supply of these beneficial herbs. These herbs are those that you commonly snip into your sauces and soups. They can also be used to soothe an itchy rash or cough. Growing medicinal herbs may not sound to be very appealing, however you can benefit from growing these plants that can provide instant relief for many illnesses that can happen anytime of the day.

It would also be wonderful to be able to cut a sprig of thyme while boiling water and prepare a fresh cup of thyme tea that is fragrant and vibrant. Since it is fresh, you'll sure it is effective since it's fresh.

So what kind of medicinal plants should you grow? The next chapter of this book features a list of different herbs and medicinal plants that you can grow at home. The list is just a good starting point for easy to find and easy to grow herbs. The same plants that you can use in cooking daily may also be used as teas, salves, washes and tinctures. You can also make cough syrup and cough drops with the very same herbal plants that you grow in the comforts of your own home.

No matter how you thoroughly care for your medicinal plants, in the long run, they will have to be replaced. If this should happen during the colder days, you will have to take into account the growing time, before they will be big enough for harvest. Commonly, this will take about 4 to 6 weeks. You can make use of these herbs not only for cooking but for medicinal purposes as well.

What problems can you possibly encounter while growing medicinal plants and herbs in your home garden? While herbs typically suffer from much less issues that flowers and vegetables do, there are a few things that should be looked out for. Plants grown in your home garden may also encounter some basic problems such as molds or mildew problems, insect damage and most of all, fertilizer issues. To remedy these problems, you must know the following guidelines:

1. Home Garden Temperature

   While most of us think our homes as a temperate area would be ideal for growing plants, this is not always the case.

   A plant requires light in order to make food, a process which we know as photosynthesis. While plants are very adaptable, they grow best within a 70 to 75 degree range. A plant utilizes more energy when the temperature is warm than when it is cold. Plants can adapt to a cooler room, for instance, with an air conditioner. The plants will begin the process of photosynthesis with the increase in temperature and there will be no sunlight to produce food. When this happens, the plants will not most likely to thrive and will probably die.

So what is the best temperature for growing medicinal herbs?

Plants grow best when there is at least a 10 degree fall in temperature during the night. During the summer, the temperature tends to get high and stay high. Plants get stressed and become highly susceptible to diseases. They grow less and can drop leaves, weaken and die, despite sufficient watering. If you are growing herbs indoors, it would be a good idea to grow them around a room based on available temperature zones. Save a lot of money and be stress-free by working on with what you already have instead of trying to make big modifications that work against the natural rhythm of your home environment.

2. Home Garden Fertilizer

Once you have already decided on which type of herbs that you will grow in your home garden, you will now have to choose the most suitable fertilizer for them. Not all fertilizers are created the same. While most have advertising claims, these fertilizers may be overused enough to damage your medicinal herbs grown at home.

What kinds of fertilizers can be used at home? There are a lot of fertilizer types that will work for your medicinal herb garden at home. For indoor plants, you can try using a variety that can be dissolved in water (water-soluble). This particular type of fertilizer may come in packaged granular form that you measure and dissolve in water prior to application. It may also come in the form of a fish emulsion, which is a concentrated variety and is combined with water before application.

Regardless on the type of fertilizer that you choose to use, you must apply it at one quarter of the packaging's recommended amount. Apply this light mixture once every week. For a more effective application, make sure to water your plants thoroughly and then apply the prepared fertilizer solution. This technique will allow for better absorption by the plant.

More importantly, make sure that you do a monthly flushing of your medicinal plants. This can be done by placing the plant in a sink and water entirely, allowing the excess water to draw off. Once the dripping stops, water completely once again. This technique will get rid of any salts that may have accumulated in the plant's soil.

Chapter 2: Easy Guide to Successfully Grow Herbs and Medicinal Plants at Home

Follow this easy step-by-step guide to start with your medicinal herb garden at home:

1. Choose your herbs. When growing medicinal herbs at home, it is important to have a good variety of herbs as well as companion plants. Some of the good choice include the following:

   - Hot pepper

   - Strawberries

   - Oregano

   - Thyme

   - Lime basil

   - Mint

   - Common basil

   - Sage

   - Lemon balm

   - Sweet marjoram

2. Prepare your pot. Be sure that the pots that you will be using for your medicinal plants have holes at the bottom to provide good drainage. With a grit or gravel, pour to about a quarter of the pot's depth. This will allow the water to steep out from the soil's bottom.

3. Fill. When the gravel is already in place, begin to fill the pot with soil-based or multi-purpose compost. Fill t about three (3) quarters of the pot's remaining space.

4. Begin planting – put the medicinal plants into the pot, with around 15 centimeters between each stem. Squeeze every plant lightly from its temporary pot. To encourage the plants to spread out, tease the roots from the root ball.

5. Put the trailing plants near the edge and the taller ones in the center of the display. This technique will endure the best growth for your plants. DO not

worry if the display may seem to appear messy at first. This will begin to fill out and look lush in just a few weeks.

6. Fill in the spaces around the plants. When you are already satisfied with the positions, begin filling in the gaps in between the plants with compost. Tightly push the compost into the spaces by pushing your fingers deep into the soil. Be careful not to injure the roots. Add more if needed. To avoid overflowing when being waters, leave a few centimeters between the rim of the pot and the soil.

7. Top the plants. Cut the taller plants' top. This will encourage them to bush out and give more fresh leaves to pick during harvest time.

8. Fertilize regularly. Purchase a controlled release fertilizer which should last a whole season. This will mean that you won't have to feed the pot again.

9. Water. Water your plants thoroughly or until the water begins to drain out of the pot's bottom. Medicinal plants usually like to dry out between watering and some types of medicinal plants such as Rosemary can easily be over-watered.

Growing herbs and medicinal plants at home is an easy yet a very rewarding hobby. Below are seven (7) key steps that will surely help you to successfully grow a healthy medicinal herb at home:

1. Keep an eye on Pests

   Medicinal herbs are generally not bothered so much about pests as much as flowers and vegetables can be. In an indoor garden however, the non-natural conditions may increase the possibility of a pest problem. To keep pests from damaging your medicinal plants in your indoor garden, make sure to keep a close eye. At the very first sight of infestation, make use of a soapy spray. You may also handpick any pests that you may have come to notices and put sticky traps to get rid of the rest.

2. Water your plants regularly

   Medicinal herbs require thorough attention when it comes to watering. Whether your medicinal plants likes drier conditions or extra moisture, it is never a good idea to have plants to be sitting in water.

3. Apply fertilizer

   Always keep in mind that medicinal plants grown indoors require a special fertilization schedule than those which are planted in an outdoor environment.

4. Be mindful of the soil

   Indoor gardening soil needs to have effective exceptional drainage. It also needs to be light. Whether your medicinal plants like drier conditions or with extra moisture, having your plants to sit in water is never a good idea. Specifically buy potting soil. You may also prepare your own by using a part of peat moss, a part of sand and a part of bagged potting soil.

5. Ensure proper circulation

   Medicinal plants require sufficient airflow to keep pests and bacterial organisms at bay. Just make sure to keep the air moving in the area where you will grow your medicinal plants.

6. Check your temperature

   Keep your planting area at constant temperature. The ideal temperature for a home garden is about 60 to 70 degrees.

7. Provide enough light

   Provide about 14 to 16 hours of artificial light to keep your medicinal plants healthy. You can also alternatively expose them to natural light for about 6 hours a day.

Chapter 3: The Best Medicinal Plants to Grow at Home

Do you have a small space at home to grow some plants? Why not grow some medicinal plants? Growing your own medicinal plants will not only get a lot of enjoyment but this will also provide medicinal relief at the comforts of your own home. While herbal remedies must never take the place of professional health care, it would be nice to have a sense of self-help should you ever end up having to need instant relief. Below is a list of the best plants to start your own personal medicinal plants garden:

1. Echinacea – this herb is also popularly known as the purple coneflower. Echinacea is an American perennial wildflower which is popularly known for its stimulating effects in the immune system. Preparations made with this wonder herb are used for the treatment of flu, colds, minor infections and a wide range of various illnesses.

2. Lavender – is medicinal plant which is commonly used as a fragrance these days. Lavender has been widely used since ancient times to reduce swelling, provide relief for rashes and itching and to treat burns, bug bites and other skin orders.

3. Lemon Balm – Prepare potent lemonade by adding bruised lemon balm leaves into your drink. This herb is commonly used as a calming "night tea" to combat insomnia. It can also make an effective topical relief for cold sores.

4. Comfrey – The roots of this wonder herb are cooked and mashed to make a potent topical relief for sprains, burns, bruises and arthritis. Just do not eat it. There is a study which reported that this herb can potentially damage the liver in eaten in significant amounts.

5. St. John's Wort – this wonder herb can lift the mood very well that you must keep from using this when you are already taking other forms of anti-depressants. The flowers and leaves of this herb may be used to prepare a tea. They can also be soaked in liquor to make a tincture. In a recent announcement, the FDA warned the public that there was a risk of adverse reactions between this herb and certain prescription drugs used for the treatment of cancer, transplant rejection, heart disease and AIDS, among others.

6. Borage – this potent herb has beautiful flowers that may be soaked in alcohol to prepare a powerful tonic that can boost your mood. The flowers and leaves may be used in tea preparations, eaten raw or soaked in liquor

or wine to flavor the drink. The fresh plant provides a salty flavor with a cucumber-like smell.

7. Peppermint – this medicinal plant can be an effective tonic to promote better digestion. However, peppermint and any other strong mints such as pennyroyal must not be taken by women who are pregnant or possibly be pregnant. Drinks and foods that have fresh strong mint leaf can be harmful to the baby.

8. Pennyroyal – just like peppermint, pennyroyal is a great smelling mint which can be crushed and topically applied to the skin as a very powerful insect repellent. The leaves of pennyroyal can be crushed and topically applied to wounds as an antiseptic agent. It can also be used in tea preparations to tame upset stomach, however, do not over do it. The maximum recommendation is 2 cups daily. Consuming more than this recommendation may cause cramps and nausea.

9. Aloe vera – is a plant native to tropical Africa. This plant has spread worldwide as a first medicinal herb that provides soothing effects for scalds and burns. Aloe vera is best grown in a container so that it can be easily transferred indoors during the winter season.

10. Yarrow – for someone who's about to start a medicinal garden at home, yarrow is usually the top pick. This herb is a beautiful perennial plant that can serve a lot of different uses. Crushed yarrow flowers and leaves may be directly applied to scratches and cuts to reduce the chances of infections and to stop bleeding.

11. Slippery Elm – the inner back of this wonder herb can be ground and made into a nutrient-rich porridge-like soup. This can be an effective remedy for sore throat. In addition to this, the inner bark of this herb can be soothe irritations in the digestive tract.

12. Fenugreek – the seeds of this medicinal plant are nourishing and used to:

- Restore a dull sense of taste
- Freshen the breath
- Ease labor pains
- Ease painful menstruation
- Help in insufficient lactation
- Promote better digestion
- Help for late onset diabetes

- Darin off sweat ducts

- Treat inflammation and ulcers of the intestines and stomach

- Reduce blood cholesterol levels

- Inhibit cancer of the liver

- Encourage weight gain

13. Feverfew – is a plant which can be made into tea for the treatment of fevers, colds and arthritis. This plant is said to have sedative properties. It can also regulate menstruation. A feverfew infusion may be used to bathe swollen feet. It can also be made into a tincture for the treatment of bruises. Chewing about 4 pieces of leaves daily has been proven to be an effective cure for some migraine headaches.

14. Comfrey – an herb which contains allantoin. This substance is a cell proliferant which boosts the natural replacement of body cells. Comfrey is widely known for its ability to build strong teeth and bones in children. Comfrey is safer to use externally than internally. This wonder herb is used to treat a wider variety of health issues including the following:

- Varicose veins

- Eczema

- Sores

- Sprains

- Bruises

- Cuts

- Acne

- Severe burns

- Varicose and gastric ulcers

- Arthritis

- Sprains

- Broken bones

- Bronchial problems

15. Milk Thistle – this powerful herb can protect and improve the function of the liver. This herb may be taken internally to help treat the following:

- The effects of a hangover

- The growth of cancer cells in prostate, cervical and breast cancer

- Insulin resistance in patients suffering from type 2 diabetes who also have cirrhosis

- Increased cholesterol levels

- Liver inflammation or hepatitis

- Jaundice

- Gall bladder diseases

- Liver diseases

16. Wu Wei Zi – the fruit of this herb are reported to stimulate the central nervous system when used in low doses. In large doses, the fruits are said to depress the central nervous system while regulating the cardiovascular system. The seeds of this herb are used in the treatment of cancer. When used externally, this herb is used to treat allergic and irritating skin problems. Internally, this herb is used to treat the following conditions:

- Diabetes

- Hepatitis

- Hyperacidity

- Poor memory

- Insomnia

- Palpitations

- Chronic diarrhea

- Involuntary ejaculation

- Urinary disorders

- Night sweats

- Asthma

- Dry coughs

17. Sage – the latin name for this herb, "salvia", means to heal. When used internally, this herb treats the following conditions:

   - Menopausal problems

   - Femal sterility

   - Depression

   - Anxiety

   - Excessive salivation

   - Excessive perspiration

   - Excessive lactation

   - Liver issues

   - Flatulence

   - Indigestion

   When used externally, sage is used for:

   - Vaginal discharge

   - Skin infections

   - Gum infections

   - Mouth infections

   - Throat infection

   - Skin infections

   - Insect bites

18. Turkey Rhubarb – this herb is popularly known for its beneficial and positive effect on the digestive system. Even children can take advantage of the beneficial effects of this herb because it is gentle enough. In low doses, the roots can serve as an astringent tonic for better digestion while higher doses may be used as laxatives. In addition to this, turkey rhubarb is also known to treat the following:

   - Skin eruptions because of toxin accumulation

- Menstrual problems

- Hemorrhoids

- Gall bladder problems

- Liver diseases

- Diarrhea

- Chronic constipation

19. Ginseng – is one of the most highly repudiated medicinal herbs in the orient. This wonder herb is touted for its ability to promote overall health, and general body vigor. The roots of this amazing medicinal plant is used to:

- Treat insomnia

- Address lack of appetite

- Treat debility related to old age

- Boost resistance against diseases

- Reduce levels of cholesterol

- Reduce blood sugar levels

- Enhance stamina

- Promote secretion of hormones

- Relax and stimulate the nervous system

20. Evening Primrose - the young roots of this medicinal plant can be consumed like a vegetable. The shoots may also be eaten as a salad. The roots of this wonder herb can be applied to bruises and piles. The roots may also be made into tea for the treatment of bowel pains and obesity. However, the more valuable parts are the bark and the leaves which are made into evening primrose oil, which is popularly known to treat the following conditions:

- Alcohol-associated liver damage

- Rheumatoid arthritis

- Brittle nails

- Acne

- Eczema

- Hyperactivity

- Premenstrual tension

- Multiple sclerosis

21. Tea tree – even the aborigines have utilized the leaves of tea tree for medicinal purposes, such as chewing fresh leaves to ease headaches. The twigs, and leaves are made into tea tree oil which has antiseptic, antibacterial and antifungal properties. Tea tree oil definitely deserves a place in every household medicine cabinet. Tea tree oil is widely used for the treatment of the following illnesses:

  - Minor burns

  - Nits

  - Cold sores

  - Insect bites

  - Warts

  - Athlete's foot

  - Acne

  - Vaginal infections

  - Thrush

  - Chronic fatigue syndrome

  - Glandular fever

  - Cystitis

22. Great yellow gentian – the root of this powerful herb which is used to treat digestive problems. It is also capable of stimulating the digestive system, gallbladder and the liver. When taken internally, it is used to treat the following conditions:

  - Anorexia

  - Gastric infections

- Indigestion
- Liver complaints

Chapter 4: Know the Ten (10) Most Common Herb and Medicinal Garden Mistakes and How to Avoid Them

Common Mistake No. 1: Not applying any fertilizers.

Once you have herbs and medicinal plants planted and growing, it is very essential to keep them growing healthy with the use of a light, all purpose fertilizer. Apply a compost tea once every week to give your herbal and medicinal plants a boost. Herbs and medicinal plants are going to be harvested a lot of times during the growing season. This only means that your plants will be need an extra boost in order to keep their growth cycle for an extended time. When applying fertilizer, make sure to keep the soil hydrated and not the leaves themselves along with the compost tea. This practice will be healthier for the plant and contaminations in the leaves will also be avoided.

Common Mistake No. 2: Not protecting the plants enough.

While the herbal and medicinal plants are known to be hardy and resistant to diseases and bug problems, they can still arise. A lot of times, herbal and medicinal plant gardeners are scared to employ any strategy to safeguard their plants. This should not be the case. There are a lot of homemade and organic controls that are safe to use for edible herbal and medicinal plants. Organic gardening begins before the plant is even in place. Good soil and beneficial insects work altogether towards a chemical free herbal and medicinal garden.

Common Mistake No. 3: Not watering the plants properly

The needs of herbal and medicinal plants are very minimal. While they are very easy to maintain and care for, these plants will be providing you with fresh harvest all season. Herbal and medicinal plants however require proper watering schedule in order to remain free from stress.

Herbal and medicinal plants should be watered in the early morning, if possible. In this way, the water will soak deeper into the soil without having to deal with any evaporation issue. Always keep the soil around the plant hydrated and never water over the leaves as this will only promote diseases and mildews. Good mulch is important for your herbs as well. This will keep the soil hydrated and may extend the time between watering. Avoid mulching right next to the plant's stem though as this may invite insects and other types of invaders to make their home.

Common Mistake No. 4: Not paying attention to the tiny details.

It is a must to watch herbal and medicinal gardens closely. You need to know what the plant should look like while it is healthy as this will allow you to immediately notice when a problem first happens. Keep an eye on any damaged stems, leaves and disturbed soil around the plant. If you notice that the stems and leaves are beginning to fade, turn brown or curl up, you will have became aware of the problem early enough to possibly save the plant.

Common Mistake No. 4: Spraying chemical compounds into the plants

Herbs and medicinal plants are usually rinsed and used fresh. They should never be exposed to any kind of treatment that may possibly be toxic or dangerous to those who would eat them.

Even if a product claims that it is safe to use around pets and people, you should look for the words safe for edibles. You cannot rinse a bunch of basil leaves with water and soup prior to using. There are a lot of ways to keep ahead of the problems that may require the application of chemicals. Weed on a regular basis, watch the plants closely for any insect infestation and use natural fertilizers such as compost tea.

Common Mistake No. 5: Allowing the flowers to turn into seeds.

Herbal and medicinal plants grow beautiful flowers. While a lot of these plants have edible flowers, it is not a great idea to allow the herb to flower early during the growing season. Once your plant flowers, this signals that its life cycle is about to come into an end. Your plant is growing a flower, then a seed, then it dies back for that particular season.

It is a better idea to keep any blossoms from forming in the first place. When you see a flower about to grow, just pinch the entire thing off. You will notice that the plant may become persistent. In such case, cut the entire stem or below the flower.

Common Mistake No. 6: overcrowding or planting incorrectly

It is common to purchase more plants that you can possibly grow in a given area. When purchasing your herbal and medicinal plants, read the plant tags that usually come with each pot. Keep an eye to the width and height of the fully grown plant. You can always grow a quick growing annual between the plants, if you do not prefer the look of mulch. It is always a good idea to underplant rather than plant the herbs too close to each other from the beginning. Over planting is a big waste for money as it will not allow your plants to grow a healthy root system. A sturdy root system will help them survive the winter and expand the next growing season.

Common Mistake No. 7: Not cutting back enough

Pruning is what makes a plant to grow fast and neat. Pruning an herb implies that you are actually harvesting the good tasting stems and leaves. If you omit pruning, the plant will only tend to grow taller on a few stems. The leaves will grow old, dry and fall off. This will result to longer stems without leaves, Pruning will also allow the plant to begin and finish its life cycle. By regular pruning, you are actually keeping the plant in its growing phase for as long as possible. It will keep the flowers from budding, promotes leaves and stems and keeps the plant producing for an extended period of time. Your plants will appear healthier and better, if pruned back on a regular basis.

Common Mistake No. 9: Growing the plants in the wrong environment.

Are you growing rosemary, a chalky and dry loving plant in a humid and moist area? Your plant will surely die off in about 2 weeks from wet feet. If you would like to grow plants in a shady area, go for plants that can tolerate less sun. The sun=loving plants will grow weak and pale from not enough bright sunlight daily. If you have neither too shady nor too sunny area, try planting in pots that can be rolled or moved to the optimal lighting conditions. It is not a matter of sufficient shading or sun but is just a matter of finding a way to be adaptable to what you already have.

Common Mistake No. 10: Choosing unhealthy medicinal and herbal plants

The very first chance you have to find the perfect plant is when you actually buy it. Search for healthy plants, bright in color, plenty of foliage and certainly not one egg or bug on it. Finding a single aphid means that there are a lot more that you cannot see, all awaiting for the perfect time to invade your other plants. Never have the sympathy for a weak looking plant, unless you have a lot of space to keep it isolated from your main garden area while you try to repair the damage. The effort and time to be spent in repairing an infested herb garden means wasted time. Take the extra step to look for the healthiest plants that you can purchase.

Conclusion

Thank you again for purchasing this book!

I hope this book was able to help you to know how to successfully grow medicinal plants and herbs at home.

The next step is to follow the step-by-step guide and see your plants grow healthier each day.

Finally, if you enjoyed this book, please take the time to share your thoughts and post a review on Amazon. We do our best to reach out to readers and provide the best value we can. Your positive review will help us achieve that. It'd be greatly appreciated!

Thank you and good luck!

Check Out My Other Books

Below you'll find some of my other popular books that are popular on Amazon and Kindle as well. Simply click on the links below to check them out. Alternatively, you can visit my author page on Amazon to see other work done by me.

Coconut Oil for Easy Weight Loss

http://amzn.to/1i5f45p

Essential Oils & Aromatherapy

http://amzn.to/1ouuZTx

Superfoods that Kickstart Your Weight Loss

http://amzn.to/1eyHdku

The Best Secrets Of Natural Remedies

http://amzn.to/1gmHd7y

The Hypothyroidism Handbook

http://amzn.to/1emWfyR

The Hyperthyroidism Handbook

http://amzn.to/1kqLQCp

Essential Oils & Weight Loss For Beginners

http://amzn.to/Q83bFp

ESSENTIAL OILS BOX SET #15: The Beginners Guide to Making Your Own Essential Oils and The Beginners Guide to Medicinal Plants

Top Essential Oil Recipes

http://amzn.to/1lSrhSC

Soap Making For Beginners

http://amzn.to/1fkmYwr

Body Butters For Beginners

http://amzn.to/1fWjwJe

Homemade Body Scrubs & Masks For Beginners

http://amzn.to/1jjLRIO

Carrier Oils For Beginners

http://amzn.to/1sbqUQP

Natural Homemade Cleaning Recipes For Beginners

http://amzn.to/1izDB2m

The Beginners Guide To Medicinal Plants

http://amzn.to/1vSujr6

The Beginners Guide To Making Your Own Essential Oils

http://amzn.to/1piUNSB

The Beginners Alkaline Miracle Diet

ESSENTIAL OILS BOX SET #15: The Beginners Guide to Making Your Own Essential Oils and The Beginners Guide to Medicinal Plants

http://amzn.to/1sDVaVE

Thyroid Diet

http://amzn.to/1piW2RY

Essential Oils Box Set #1 (Weight Loss + Essential Oil Recipes

http://amzn.to/1qlYWWP

Essential Oils Box Set #2 (Weight Loss + Essential Oil & Aromatherapy

http://amzn.to/1qlYWWP

Essential Oils Box Set #3 Coconut Oil + Apple Cider Vinegar

http://amzn.to/1oIFZJw

Essential Oils Box Set #4 Body Butters & Top Essential Oil Recipes

http://amzn.to/1jSxURJ

Essential Oils Box Set #5 Soap Making & Homemade Body Scrubs

http://amzn.to/RAvJYo

Essential Oils Box Set #6 Body Butters & Body Scrubs

http://amzn.to/RAvSel

Essential Oils Box Set #7 Top Essential Oils & Best Kept Secrets Of Natural Remedies

http://amzn.to/1gvsRCq

ESSENTIAL OILS BOX SET #15: The Beginners Guide to Making Your Own Essential Oils and The Beginners Guide to Medicinal Plants

Essential Oils Box Set #8 Homemade Cleaning Recipes & Essential Oil Recipes

http://amzn.to/1gxFAVb

Essential Oils Box Set #9 Essential Oil and Weight Loss & Carrier Oils

http://amzn.to/1jmcEPP

Essential Oils Box Set #10 Hyperthyroidism Manual & Hypothyroidism Manual

http://amzn.to/1nHgJU4

Essential Oils Box Set #11 Carrier Oils for Beginners & Coconut Oil for Easy Weight Loss

http://amzn.to/1nHfy6X

Essential Oils Box Set #12 Essential Oils Weight Loss & Essential Oils Aromatherapy & Natural Homemade Cleaning Supplies & Top Essential Oil Recipes & Carrier Oils
http://amzn.to/1nHfy6X

Essential Oils Box Set #13 Superfoods & Essential Weight Loss & Essential Aromatherapy & Body Butters & Soap Making
http://amzn.to/1nUds6v

Essential Oils Box Set #14 Weight Loss & Apple Cider Vinegar & Body Butters & Homemade Body Scrubs & Coconut Oil for Beginners
http://amzn.to/1i1qYOd

If the links do not work, for whatever reason, you can simply search for these titles on the Amazon website to find them.